John ‹

Perioperative Topics:
Test and Learn

Table of Contents

Disclaimer

The author has made every effort to ensure that the contents of this book are correct, error free, and a reasonable representation of the design goal, which is to provide the reader with a non-stressful means of assessing their personal knowledge, strengths, and weaknesses, with respect to some of the general principles of effective perioperative health care.

The author accepts no responsibility or liability for damages caused by any erroneous contents of this book and, in all situations, recommends that professional guidelines, national policies, and direction from suitably qualified medical staff, take precedence over the information contained herein.

duplicated or distributed in any form, without written permission from the author.

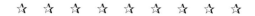

Preface

Working in the healthcare setting requires, arguably, two types of knowledge or ability.

The first type can be considered that which is accumulated through practice and experience and, in the main, concerns the practical aspects of the job in hand. As a general rule, a practitioner, such as a nurse or paramedic, for example, who has perhaps twenty years experience, will almost certainly have accumulated significantly more practical experience than another practitioner with, say, only two years experience.

The second type of ability is determined by education and investigation, and which requires specific application and research, either as part of a formal education regime, or realised in a more personal and self-directed model of learning. Unlike with the situation relating to practical experience, technical and academic abilities are not so dependent on time served undertaking the individual's particular job role; instead, it is determined more by either prior education, ongoing personal technical education and development, or a combination of both factors.

Perioperative Topics: Test and Learn, is comprised of questions (with answers) concerning a combination of both practical matters, such as knowing how pregnancy effects *Functional Residual Capacity*, and questions which can be regarded as a little more technical, such as being able to convert pressure values between millimetres of mercury and pascals.

The tests are not to be considered pass or fail. Instead, they should be seen as indicators of those areas in which the reader might require more study. Additionally, by mastering the subject matter in these (and similar) tests, the reader will assume a more confident frame of mind, particular with respect to attempting courses of study which might lead to career advancement.

Introduction

This collection of questions is loosely grouped into the categories of:

√ Emergencies

√ Basic science

√ Biology

√ Pharmacology

√ Respiration & Circulation

√ Anaesthetics

√ Monitoring

√ Surgery

• **Emergencies** includes questions on the recognition and immediate actions relating to common emergency conditions, with the emphasis on symptom recognition.

• **Basic Science**, is a short test of the reader's understanding of selected basic physics concepts, with specific inclusion of questions regarding pressure and the atmosphere, electrical safety, surgical equipment, and applicable terminology.

• **Biology** questions concern a mixture of relevant subjects, such as: anatomy, physiology, pathology, and patient conditions which require immediate recognition and action.

• **Pharmacology** focuses on a few of the main drug classifications, terminology, pharmacodynamics, and uses of selected agents for emergency situations.

• **Respiration & Circulation** concerns airway management, the respiratory process, transfusions, and infusions.

• **Anaesthetics** concerns factors which are specific to the anaesthetic function, and more general anaesthetic related factors which all healthcare practitioners should be familiar with, particularly with respect to the airway and breathing.

- **Monitoring** example topics include respiration, circulation, fluid balance, blood glucose, and post surgical care.

- **Surgery** concerns fundamental, terminology and principles.

All of the questions are accompanied by answers, some of which also include brief explanations, where appropriate, and the reader is encouraged to expand upon those explanations and answers, through further research and self-directed learning.

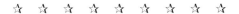

Emergencies

Soomcg   1: 1000 W\Y so\man

Asphyxia Insufficiency of O_2 in the brain'

E 1. What is an *anaphylactic shock*?

A severe reaction to a substance, such as drugs, bee stings, or peanuts, which can lead to asphyxia, cardiovascular collapse, and cardiac arrest. Intramuscular adrenaline (epinephrine) is the usual immediate treatment - 500 microgram of a 1 in 1,000 w/v solution.

E 2. Which of the following (9) are some of the signs of anaphylaxis?

a) Abdominal pain

b) Feeling faint

c. Itchy skin

d. Raised, red skin rash

e. Swollen eyes, lips, hands, feet

f. Urticaria

g. Agitation

h. Hypertension

j. Nausea and vomiting

k. Swelling of the throat and tongue

l. Unconsciousness

m. Expiratory wheeze

Answer: a, b, d, e, f, g, k, l, m.

E 3. What is a *pneumothorax*?

Gas - usually air - trapped inside the pleural cavity (between a lung and the chest wall) which may result in lung collapse. Symptoms include chest pain and tightness, tachycardia, sweating, and cyanosis. If small, treatment may not be necessary. Otherwise, the gas may have to be drained – by a chest tube, or with needle aspiration (thoracocentesis), through the second intercostal space.

E 4. What is the difference between *cardiac arrest* and *heart attack*?

Cardiac arrest is when the heart stops beating (electrical malfunction); *Heart attack* is when blood flow to a part of the heart muscle is impaired, causing ischaemia, which can result in death of the effected part of the heart.

E 5. How are the different types of sepsis differentiated?

Type	*Typical Indications*
Sepsis	Tachypnoea, tachycardia, infection, temperature < 36°, or > 38°, low BP, confusion, cyanosis
Severe sepsis	Chills, patchy skin, lethargy, low platelets, organ failure
Septic shock	As severe sepsis, + lactate > 2 mmol/L

E 6. Is it safe to use an Automated External Defibrillator on a patient who is lying on a wet surface?

There is no published evidence to prove that lying on a wet surface is a danger to patients. The AHA (American Heart Association) stipulate that the patient should be moved to a dry area, before defibrillation. However, they do not state what should be done if there is no dry surface available, or how to proceed if the patient may have spinal injury. There have been cases of successful defibrillation on patients who were lying on wet surfaces, and no reports of untoward cases.

E 7. What are the symptoms of Atrial Fibrillation? /Fast Heart beat / Irregular

☞ Arrhythmia   Abnormal Heart beat

☞ Tachycardia (often)

☞ Dizziness

☞ Palpitations (Heart pounding)

☞ Confusion

☞ Fatigue

☞ Shortness of breath

E 8. What is an embolus?

A mass, such as fat, gas, or blood, which travels around the bloodstream, and which can stop at a vessel, thereby impeding blood flow. Once stopped, it blocks its containing vessel, and becomes an *embolism*, which should be treated as an emergency, and which requires immediate expert aid.

E 9. What are the symptoms of *hypovolaemia*?

Answer:

- ☞ Pale skin
- ☞ Increased respiratory rate
- ☞ Sweating
- ☞ Hypotension
- ☞ Anxiety
- ☞ Reduced urine output

E 10. What is *Congestive Heart Failure*?

The ventricle(s) cannot pump enough blood, leading to fluid in the lungs, abdomen, liver, and lower extremities. Causes include coronary heart disease, hypertension, diabetes mellitus, or dysfunctioning heart valves.

When the Heart is unable to pump blood around the body.

14

E 11. What is the name of the condition where fluid accumulates in the pericardium faster than the pericardial sac can stretch, potentially preventing the ventricles from filling properly.

Cardiac Tamponade. Symptoms include tachycardia, anxiety, weak pulse, pain (chest, neck, back, shoulders), hypotension, muffled heart sounds, distended neck veins, and a tendency to lean forward.

E 12. How is the mean blood pressure calculated?

Blood pressure monitors use integral calculus to derive MAP (mean arterial pressure), but a good approximation can be made by adding diastolic to 1/3 pulse pressure.

E 13. What are the main types of *stroke*?

[handwritten: thickening / hardening of Artery / caused by build up of plaque]

Ischaemic: (Most common type) Blood supply to the brain is blocked, by atherosclerosis or an embolic clot. If the clot is formed in a blood vessel in the brain, the stroke is termed *thrombotic*.

Haemorrhagic: A blood vessel in the brain ruptures,

[handwritten: ischemia is insufficient blood flow to provide adequate oxygenation. This in turn leads to Hypoxia (reduced O₂) / ANOXIA (absence of O₂)]

and the leaking blood causes pressure, which can lead to cell damage.

E 14. What is a *Thrombosis*?

A clot, such as caused by plaque (atherosclerosis), which forms inside a blood vessel, impeding circulation. If part of the thrombus breaks away, it becomes an embolus.

E 15. What is the immediate management of acid reflux?

Answer:

- ☞ Head down position (Trendelenburg).

- ☞ Suction the oropharynx.

- ☞ 100% oxygen.

- ☞ Cricoid pressure.

- ☞ Rapid sequence induction.

- ☞ Suction the trachea.

- ☞ Positive End Expiratory Pressure (5 cm/H2O).

E 16. What term describes the situation where the patient's heart does not produce any electrical or mechanical activity?

Asystole (no heart contractions), and illustrated by no ECG activity. Asystole is a cardiac emergency, which requires immediate chest compressions, and compliance with the life support algorithm.

E 17. What is the definition of *post-partum haemorrhage*?

PPH is the loss of at least 500 ml (cc) of blood, from the mother, within 24 hours of giving birth. PPH is the world's primary cause of a ¼ of maternal deaths. There is conflicting evidence concerning the efficacy of tranexamic acid for managing PPH.

E 18. What is the name of the condition where there is fluid build up in the pleural space, external to the lungs?

Pleural effusion, commonly caused by, for example, pulmonary embolism, or heart failure. Primary treatment is to treat the underlying cause. A significant effusion may require intervention by aspiration with a needle, or tube through the chest.

E 19. What are the main indications for sepsis?

Answer, adults:

℣ Feeling feint	℣ Temperature above 38.3º C
℣ Muscle pain	℣ Temperature below 36º C
℣ Tachycardia	℣ Tachypnoea
℣ Chills, fever	℣ Feeling feint
℣ Muscle pain	

Children:

Similar to adults, but also with pain, nausea, and cold peripheries.

E 20. Define *Hypovolaemic Shock*.

Reduction of 15% intravascular volume, requiring immediate fluid administration, to re-establish circulating volume.

E 21. What is the definition of *Septic Shock*?

The inflammatory response to sepsis, characterised by:

⚲ Hypotension, to which fluid administration is ineffective.

⚲ Vasopressors have to be used to maintain a mean arterial pressure of at least 65 mmHg.

⚲ A serum lactate level greater than 2 mmol/litre.

Symptoms include:

Anxiety ✦ *Fatigue* ✦ *Diarrhoea* ✦ *Nausea, vomiting* ✦ *Fever* ✦ *Chills* ✦ *Muscular pain* ✦ *Breathing difficulties* ✦ *Clammy skin* ✦ *Unconsciousness*

E 22. What is the difference between an *Open* and a *Closed* Pneumothorax?

Open: air enters the chest cavity through a hole in the chest, from the environment, as occurs with penetrating injury, resulting in an equalising of pressure between the lung and atmosphere.

Closed: air enters the chest cavity (pleural space) from a hole in the lung, which tends to create a back pressure against the lung.

E 23. What are the symptoms of *malignant hyperthermia*?

  ☞ Tachycardia

  ☞ Increased CO_2 production

  ☞ Respiratory and metabolic acidosis

  ☞ Hyperventilation

  ☞ Muscle rigidity

E 24. Hypotension and tachycardia can be indicators for aspiration of gastric contents; True or false?

True; plus laryngospasm, low oxygen saturation, laryngospasm, bronchospasm, coughing.

E 25. Warfarin can be used for the immediate treatment of a deep vein thrombosis; True or false?

False; Heparin is used in the first instance - it has a quicker onset of action than Warfarin.

E 26. To counter severe hypotension, elevate the legs, tilt the bed head down, and administer fluids; True or false?

True. A vasoconstrictor (Metaraminol, Ephedrine) may also be given.

E 27. What is the recommended scalpel size for an emergency cricothyrotomy?

A size 10 blade is used to make a vertical incision, about 1.6 inch (4 cm) long. The incision must be central (medial), so that anatomical components, such as the vagus nerve, internal jugular vein, and common carotid artery are not damaged. Once the cricothyroid membrane can be palpated (felt), the scalpel is rotated 90, and then punctures the cricothyroid membrane.

E 28. What is *tension pneumothorax*?

Pneumothorax where air builds up in the pleural cavity, and has no place to diffuse to (equalise with) so, like a balloon, the pressure increases and, consequently, the pressure presses against, or collapses, the adjacent lung.

E 29. One immediate treatment for anaphylactic shock is intravenous crystalloid; True or false?

True. Fluid administration helps compensate for fluid leaking from the circulation, and mitigates against hypotension. (Note: oxygen is also advised.)

E 30. What are the initial signs of local anaesthetic toxicity?

☞ Tinnitus ☞ Sudden agitated manner

☞ Convulsions ☞ Twitching

☞ Arrhythmias ☞ Sinus bradycardia

☞ Unconsciousness ☞ Numbness (mouth, tongue)

E 31. What are the main signs that a pregnant patient has pre-eclampsia?

Answer:

- ✦ High blood pressure

- ✦ Protein in the urine

- ✦ Fluid retention

(Algorithms and treatment packs must be available in clinical obstetric areas)

E 32. What is *Right Heart Failure*?

A congestive condition where blood engorges the systemic veins, due to pulmonary hypertension, or fluid accumulation in other parts of the body, such as the abdominal cavity or skin, resulting in a failure to complete the return circuit of the blood, to the lungs.

E 33. What is *Left Heart Failure*?

Inability of the left ventricle to produce sufficient cardiac output of oxygenated blood, into the systemic circulation. Symptoms: fatigue, dizziness, confusion.

E 34. What does *pericardiocentesis* refer to?

The aspiration of fluid (pericardial effusion, or cardiac tamponade) from the pericardium, through the fifth intercostal space, typically, under sedation.

E 35. The pooling of blood in the pleural space is known as...?

1. Pneumothorax
2. Cardiac tamponade
3. Haemothorax
4. Pleurisy

Answer: 3 - Haemothorax, an instance of which is called a *haemothorace*, and is usually caused by a blunt or penetrating trauma to the chest.

E 36. What are the two most common causes of tracheal deviation?

✦ Tension pneumothorax: **deviation from** the (low pressure) pneumothorax to the opposite side. Treatment is needle aspiration to second intercostal space.

✦ Lobar collapse: **deviation towards** the collapse.

Other causes: pulmonary fibrosis, pleural fibrosis, atelectasis, pneumonectomy, pleyral effusion, mediastinal lymphoma.

E 37. Propofol or thiopentone may be given to control seizures associated with local anaesthetic systemic toxicity; True or false?

True (given in small doses). Also, benzodiazepines.

E 38. List some of the signs of bronchospasm in an anaesthetised (IPPV) patient.

☞ Increased peak airway pressure

☞ Wheeze

☞ Prolonged expiration

☞ Shark fin capnograph

Treatment may be with bronchodilators, or steroids.

E 39. A diabetic coma is caused by ...

1. Hyperglycaemia

2. Hypoglycaemia

3. Hyperglycaemia or hypoglycaemia

4. Neither hyperglycaemia nor hypoglycaemia

Answer 3: Diabetic coma can be the result of hyperglycaemia or hypoglycaemia.

E 40. What do fever, tachycardia, tachypnoea, and chills suggest?

These are early signs of sepsis, and require immediate response with the **Sepsix Six**:

✔ Administer oxygen

✔ Take bloods

- ✔ Give IV antibiotics

- ✔ Give fluids

- ✔ Check lactates, haemoglobin

- ✔ Measure urine output

E 41. Name the different types of shock.

❤ Anaphylactic	❤ Cardiogenic
❤ Insulin	❤ Distributive
❤ Septic	❤ Hypovolaemic
❤ Obstructive	❤ Neurogenic

E 42. An agonal rhythm is an emergency; True or false?

True, it is a cardiac emergency, and the resuscitation algorithm for asystole should be followed.

E 43. A tightness and heavy strangling feeling, in the chest, is a sign of?

1. Pneumothorax

2. Angina

3. Bronchospasm

4. Tracheal deviation

Answer 2 – Angina, which is usually due to narrowing of arteries caused by atherosclerosis. Treated with GTN (glycerine trinitrate). *Angina Pectoris*: Cardiac pain, caused by insufficient blood supply to the heart. *Unstable Angina:* A less predictable and less controllable from of angina.

E 44. Define APGAR.

A rating method to quickly assess the health of new born children, based on **appearance, pulse, grimace, activity**, and **respiration**.

E 45. What is the name of the congestive heart condition where not enough blood is returned from the venal system, to the right heart, causing pulmonary congestion,, systemic venal congestion and oedema.

Answer: Backward Heart Failure.

E 46. Why is a Urea and Electroly
during a cardiac arrest?

A "U and Es" report shows what irregularities might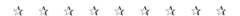
contributory or reversible causes of the arrest,
particularly regarding potassium, calcium, sodium,
bicarbonate, and glucose. Metabolic disorders might also
reveal underlying problems with kidney function, and
reveal causes of acid-base imbalance.

E 47. What does a VIP Score of 5 mean?

Thrombophlebitis at the site of a peripheral cannula,
which requires treatment and resiting of the cannula.

E 48. Is *Insulin Shock* caused by too much or too little
insulin?

Too much: perhaps due to injecting too much insulin,
causing hypoglycaemia.

☆ ☆ ☆ ☆ ☆ ☆ ☆ ☆ ☆

Basic Science

G 1. What is the mean pressure of air at mean sea level and standard temperature?

Standard Pressure is 1 atm (atmosphere), and is equivalent to 760 mmHg, or 101.325 kPa. Standard temperature is 273 K (0° C, or 32° Fahrenheit).

G 2. What does *anodyne* refer to?

A pain relieving drug.

G 3. How are Pascals related to Newtons?

A Pascal is an S.I. (Système Internationale) derived unit

of pressure, defined as one Newton of force applied over one square metre. When applying cricoid pressure, during a rapid sequence induction, 30 Newtons is regarded as the amount of force required to occlude the oesophagus.

G 4. What is the function of the *Pin Index System*?

To ensure that high pressure gas cylinders are fitted to their appropriate gas mating yokes, thereby preventing coupling of cylinders to incorrect gas lines.

G 5. At what level does electrical current become painful?

10 milliamp, for a normally healthy adult. A lethal current is ~ 30 milliamp. If an electrical supply has a voltage of 50 volt or less, the severity of shock (current) is deemed unlikely to cause death, unless the patient's skin has very low resistance, such as when it is wet; which is why some medical devices have transformers, which reduce the supplied voltage to a 50 volt level.

G 6. Define *diffusion*?

The passive (no energy required) movement of molecules or other particles along a concentration gradient - from regions of higher to lower concentration. Also called migration; an intermingling of molecules, ions, etc., resulting from random thermal agitation, as in the dispersion of a vapour in air, or movement of oxygen from the alveoli to the surrounding capillaries.

G 7. What is an *osmole*?

The osmole (osmol) describes the number of moles of solute which contribute to the osmotic pressure of a solution. For example, when one mole of NaCl (sodium chloride) dissolves in water, it dissociates into one mole each of sodium and chlorine. (The dissociation of NaCl occurs because it is an ionic molecule, which produces a relatively weak bond.)

G 8. What is the mean partial pressure of oxygen, in atmospheric air, at mean sea level, and at standard temperature?

Approximately 21 kPa (160 mmHg).

G 9. Air is a fluid; True or false?

True; it flows, and does not have a fixed shape. Note that gases and liquids are both fluid.

G 10. At the summit of Mt Everest, oxygen makes up $\cong$ 21% of ambient air; True or false?

True. There are fewer gas molecules, but the proportion of oxygen, in the air, is the same as that at sea level.

G 11. A *molar* solution means there is one mole of solute per kg of solution; True or false?

False; One mole per *litre* of solution, which is a **molarity** of one.

G 12. Explain what S.I. means.

Système International d'Unités - the standard set of seven measurement systems, from which, other systems, such as pressure (pascal), are derived:

Dimension	Unit
Length	Metre
Mass	Kilogram
Time	Second
Electrical current	Ampere
Temperature	Kelvin
Amount of a substance	Mole
Light intensity	Candela

G 13. What is the meaning of the prefix *supra*?

Above or over something, such as in *supra-glottic airway device* (laryngeal mask airway), which sits above (or next to) the glottis.

G 14. What is an *emetogenic* substance?

One which causes nausea or vomiting. Opioids, for example, have the side-effect of being emetogenic.

G 15. Carbon dioxide represents approximately 5% of expired air; True or false?

True. At *Standard Pressure*, the partial pressure is approximately 38 mmHg, or 5 kPa, which is 5% of one standard atmosphere (760 mmHg, 101 kPa).

G 16. What is the effect of breathing oxygen at elevated partial pressures?

Oxygen toxicity, with symptoms:

- Disorientation
- Vision problems
- Anxiety
- Vomiting
- Burning sensation when deep breathing

G 17. What is *recrudescence*?

The resumption of a condition, or symptoms, some days after a period of remission.

G 18. Define *Molality*.

The number of moles of solute per mass (kg) of solution. If 1 kg of a solution contains 2 moles of solute, the solution molality is 2.

G 19. What is the difference between weight and mass?

Mass can be thought of as a measurement of resistance to changes in inertia, measured in kilograms (S.I.), and is the same on Earth as it is in the micro-gravity of space.

Weight represents the force exerted on a mass, measured in Newtons, and changes according to whatever local fields, such as gravity, the mass is subject to.

G 20. Carbon is the most abundant element in the body, by mass; True or false;

False; Oxygen makes up 65% of the total; carbon comprises only 18%.

G 21. Electric current is measured in *volts*; True or false?

False, current is measured in *amperes*. Voltage measures potential difference of electromotive force. Electrical danger is not directly determined by voltage level – it is the level of current, and the length of exposure, which determines the severity of electrocution.

G 22. Convert 120 mmHg to pascals.

One atmosphere is 760 mmHg, or 101 kPa (rounded). 120 mmHg is a 120/760 = 0.158 fraction of an atmosphere, therefore, 120 mmHg is equal to 0.158 * 101 = 15.9 kPa.

G 23. If a patient is given a fluid which is termed *isotonic*, how does that affect the cells?

Isotonic substances have the same osmotic pressure, so the fluid will not cause, by itself, any exchange of fluid between intracellular and interstitial spaces – the cells will not gain or lose fluid due to the administered isotonic fluid. 0.9% weight/volume sodium chloride is said to be isotonic with body fluids.

G 24. What does *aetiology* refer to?

The study of the causes of disease.

G 25. A pressure of 760 mmHg is equivalent to 1 kilopascal (kPa); True or false?

False; 760 mmHg is equivalent to 101.325 kPa.

G 26. Helium is classed as an explosive gas; True or false?

False; Helium is non-toxic, and inert (inactive).

G 27. If an oxygen cylinder is stored next to a source of heat, the increasing temperature will increase the oxygen pressure; True or false?

True; with a fixed volume, the cylinder contents must obey Boyle's Law, where *pressure * volume = temperature * number of moles * gas constant*. {The same situation occurs in weather reports, where increased air pressure is associated with increased air temperature.}

G 28. How is an electrolyte formed?

When a substance (solute) is dissolved in water, where it dissociates into its respective ions, which are negatively charged **anions**, and positively charged **cations**. The resulting solution is then electrically conductive.

G 29. If a substance, such as a drug, has a metabolic half life of two hours, how long will it take for 7/8 of the substance to be metabolised?

Answer: Six hours...

2 hours to metabolise ½ of the substance,

4 hours to metabolise ½ of the remainder - leaving ¼,

6 hours to metabolise ½ of the remainder – leaving ⅛.

G 30. What does the term "afferent" refer to?

a. From the peripheral to the centre

b. From the centre to the peripheral

c. No direction

Answer: a, from the periphery to the centre.

G 31. What does the term "affinity" refer to?

The degree to which one substance binds with another, forming a chemical compound, such as the affinity of a drug molecule to bind with its target receptor.

G 32. What significance to patient monitoring is an "artefact"?

An artefact is something which is artificially introduced, by human intervention, and may produce misleading results. A typical artefact is what appears with ECG traces, when diathermy is used on a patient – the trace looks chaotic.

G 33. What absolute gas pressure is typically delivered to an anaesthetic machine?

   a. 1 bar

   b. 5 bar

   c. 21 bar

   d. 101 bar

Answer: b, 5 bar absolute, or 4 bar relative.

G 34. If a neutrally charged atom loses an electron, what entity is formed?

A positively charged ion, known as a *cation*, because the atom now has more positive components (protons) than negative components (electrons). When an essential mineral, such as sodium or potassium, dissolves in a fluid (water), it dissociates (splits) into positively or negatively charged ions, referred to as electrolytes. These electrolytes allow electrical conduction, and make possible the body's internal communication system – nerve conduction.

G 35. A patient has an *occult* fracture; in this context, what does *occult* mean?

There are no obvious signs of the fracture, and it may not be discernible by X-ray.

G 36. What significance does a *Partition Coefficient* have to the perioperative patient?

A partition coefficient describes the ratio of concentration of a substance between two immiscible (one does not absorb the other) phases, having equal volume, pressure, and temperature. The *blood:gas partition coefficient* of a volatile inhalational agent, such as sevoflurane, which is 0.65, shows how its concentration in the blood (liquid phase) will be 0.65 of the concentration in the alveolar space (gas phase). The significance lies in the fact that an agent with a low partition coefficient will act more quickly than an agent with a higher coefficient. Comparing Isoflurane's coefficient of 1.4, with Sevoflurane's coefficient of 0.65, explains why Sevoflurane is quicker acting than Isoflurane – it is less soluble, so less of it is absorbed by the blood, which allows the alveolar and brain concentrations to build more quickly.

G 37. In an aqueous solution, the dissolved solvent is hydrophobic; True or false?

False; the solvent must be hydrophilic, otherwise it

would not be dissolved by the solvent.

G 38. If a patient receives something which originated from themselves, how is it termed?

Autologous. An example is a transplantation from one part of the patient's body to another part.

G 39. What substance is added to sterile water to extend its storage life?

Isotonic (0.9%) benzyl alcohol, a *bacteriostatic* agent, which prevents bacteria from reproducing. A *water for injections* solvent, which contains a bacteriostatic agent, is known as bacteriostatic water.

G 40. What distinguishes a colloid from a crystalloid?

A colloid is a "mixture" where one substance, with particle size between 1 and 1,000 nanometre, is evenly dispersed throughout a second substance, forming a new substance – a colloid. A crystalloid is similar, but the particle size is less than one nanometre, and can pass through the semi-permeable membrane of a capillary cell, whereas the larger colloid particles cannot, so remains within the vascular space.

G 41. What is the purpose of an *assay*?

To analyse a substance, such as blood, to determine its constituent parts, such as hormones and antibodies.

G 42. What term describes transfer of energy from glucose to cells, in the absence of oxygen?

Anaerobic Respiration. In *aerobic respiration*, moleculer oxygen (O_2) helps break down glucose, in mitochondria, converting to chemical energy (ATP) for the cell, and the waste by-products of water and carbon dioxide. In *anaerobic respiration*, energy production occurs without oxygen, and gives off lactic acid as a by-product. The lactic acid (lactate) level can be seen on arterial blood gas reports, and can help indicate ventilation problems.

Biology

B 1. If the left heart is associated with the *systemic circulation*, what is the right heart associated with?

Pulmonary circulation: the circuit between the right side of the heart, and the lungs, including pulmonary veins and arteries. The pulmonary circulation takes deoxygenated blood to the lungs, to exchange its CO_2 for oxygen, then takes the oxygenated blood to the left side of the heart, where it joins the systemic circulation.

B 2. Define *Functional Residual Capacity*?

The volume of gas remaining in the lungs after a passive expiration, which is the sum of the *expiratory reserve volume* and the *residual volume*. FRC is the lung oxygen store which, typically, is 30 mL/kg.

B 3. Functional Residual Capacity is reduced by pregnancy; True or false?

True. Also, obesity, general anaesthesia, supine and head down positions.

B 4. *Functional Residual Capacity* increases when lying down; True or false?

False; FRC reduces when lying down. That is one of the reasons why a post anaesthetic patient is placed in the sitting up position.

B 5. Mean arterial pressure is dependent on *cardiac output* and what other factor?

Mean arterial pressure =

Systemic vascular resistance * Cardiac output

B 6. What is a *surgical anastomosis*?

A connection between two hollow structures, such as two blood vessels, or two intestinal sections. If a blood vessel is blocked, the surgeon will bypass the blocked section with an anastomosis, which can be either an artificial "tubular" component, or a section of blood vessel taken from another part of the patient's body. If it is a part of the intestinal system which is blocked or damaged, the effected part will be excised (resectioned), and the two "good" ends will be anastomosed (connected).

B 7. What are typical treatments for *Deep Vein Thrombosis*?

Anticoagulation therapy (typically Heparin), walking, or Inferior Vena Cava filtration.

B 8. What is *abdominal splinting*?

A rigid contraction of the abdominal wall muscles, typically resulting from postoperative pain, which can produce hypoventilation.

B 9. What is the function of the *visceral pleura*?

It is the serous membrane which covers and protects (cushions) the lungs. Note: **Visceral** refers to *internal organs*; S**erous** means *derived from serum;* **Membrane** is a thin layer of tissues which envelopes or partitions structures.

B 10. When blood glucose levels are low, what does *glucagon* do?

Glucagon (pancreatic hormone) signals the liver to break down *glycogen* (carbohydrate, stored mostly in the liver) into *glucose*, for release into the bloodstream. This process is part of the homeostatic mechanism.

B 11. During the blood clotting process, *Thrombin* converts fibrin into fibrinogen; True or false?

False; Thrombin (factor IIa) is an enzyme which converts fibrinogen into fibrin, for use in coagulation. Additionally, it activates platelets and the coagulant factors V, VIII, XI, and XIII.

B 12. What is the term to describe the case where alveoli are perfused but not properly ventilated?

Pulmonary Shunt; Causes include pulmonary oedema and pneumonia.

B 13. What is the name of the substance which communicates messages between neurons, or between neurons and muscle fibres?

Neurotransmitter; A particular type of neurotransmitter will only bind to particular receptors. Acetylcholine (parasympathetic system), for example, binds to muscarinic and nicotinic receptors.

B 14. What structure surrounds, lubricates, and protects the heart?

The *pericardium*; a four layered structure, comprising, from the inside:

  ⚲ Visceral pericardium (serous), which covers the heart.

  ⚲ Pericardial cavity, containing pericardial fluid, to

lubricate between the visceral and parietal pericardia.

⚱ Parietal pericardium (serous membrane).

⚱ Fibrous pericardium; connective tissue to hold the heart in place, and provide mechanical protection.

B 15. *Thrombocyte* is another name for a white cell; True or false?

False; Thrombocyte is another name for a platelet. A white blood cell is a *leukocyte*.

B 16. Explain *Acid Reflux*, and its risk factors.

Stomach acid, rising up the oesophagus, from the stomach, through a faulty muscle - the *lower oesophageal sphincter*. If stomach acids find their way into the lungs, the consequences, such as aspiration pneumonia, can be severe.

Risk factors include:

☠ Non-fasted patient

☠ Bowel obstruction

- ☠ Raised intra-abdominal pressure

- ☠ Previous gastric surgery

- ☠ Hiatus hernia

- ☠ Peptic ulcers

- ☠ Pregnancy

- ☠ Old age

- ☠ Nasogastric tube in situ

- ☠ Reduced level of consciousness

- ☠ Drugs (Opiates, Volatile agents)

B 17. What is *alveolar ventilation*?

The amount of breathing gas which enters the alveoli, and is available for gas exchange. The remaining portion of gas is *deadspace* gas, especially that which does not leave the conducting zone of the respiratory tract.

B 18. What is the function of the *parasympathetic* nervous system?

It is responsible for the automatic "rest and digest"

element of the nervous system. Which includes salivation, lacrimation, arousal, digestion, waste excretion, and heart rate.

B 19. What is the name of the semi-permeable membrane which separates the blood from the brain (cerebrospinal fluid), and which protects the brain from undesirable substances, such as certain drugs, bacteria, and hormones.

The *blood brain barrier*. For a drug to do it work, it must pass the blood brain barrier – a great topic of pharmaceutical research is developing such transport mechanisms.

B 20. What is the name of the receptors which trigger cholinergic signals, in response to the binding of acetylcholine (neurotransmitter), producing slowing of the heart rate, muscle contraction, and glandular secretions.

Muscarinic, which is one of two types of (cholinergic) receptor for acetylcholine, the other being *nicotinic*.

B 21. What are the main causes of *oedema*?

Immobility, Varicose veins, Right heart failure, Pregnancy, Deep Vein Thrombosis, Allergy, Blood clots, Renal or Liver dysfunction, Obesity.

B 22. What is the name of the volume of blood expelled by the left ventricle, in one contraction?

Stroke Volume, which is typically 60-70% of the blood in the ventricle – about 2 mL/kg at rest. Stroke volume multiplied by heart rate produces *cardiac output*.

B 23. What are the main risk factors for pressure ulcers?

Dehydration; Illness; Malnutrition; Vascular disease; Extremes of age; Sensory impairment; Reduced mobility.

B 24. What is the name of the space internal to blood vessels or lymphatic ducts?

The *intravascular* space, or the space inside the blood vessels. *Extravascular* space is outside of those vessels.

B 25. Blood is comprised of platelets, red cells, white cells, and what other component?

Plasma, which represents 55% of blood volume.

B 26. What is the definition of *Perfusion*?

A liquid (e.g., oxygenated blood) passing through a vessel, or over an organ. In the body, perfusion delivers oxygen to the tissue capillaries and organs.

B 27. At rest, what is the adult normal/typical level of expired CO_2 (carbon dioxide)?

Approximately 5% of volume, or 5 kPa partial pressure. The CO_2 level increases as cardiac output increases.

B 28. What is *V/Q ratio*?

It is the ventilation/perfusion volume ratio, or the volume of air reaching the alveoli, divided by the volume of blood reaching the lungs. Normal values are 5/5 L, giving a ratio of 1. However, because ventilation and perfusion change, with respect to different parts of the lung, 0.8 is a more typical mean V/Q ratio.

B 29. Which is more likely to stimulate a higher rate of breathing, a reduction or an increase in inspired CO_2?

Increased CO_2 – it produces a respiratory drive to flush out the excess CO_2.

B 30. What is the *Vallecula*?

In the airway, the Vallecula is a furrow, between the base of the tongue and the epiglottis, which serves to prevent the constant triggering of the swallowing reflex, by acting as a spit trap.

B 31. A low level of CO_2 (carbon dioxide) in the blood, indicates an acidic condition; True or false?

False; high CO_2 means an acid condition.

B 32. All veins carry de-oxygenated blood. True or false?

False; Veins carry de-oxygenated blood, except the pulmonary veins, which transport oxygenated blood from the lungs to the left atrium. By definition, a vein carries blood towards the heart, and an artery takes blood away, regardless of oxygenation levels.

B 33. What is the *carina*?

The point at which the Trachea divides into the right and left main bronchi. It is a significant landmark in intubation.

B 34. What is the action of *acetylcholinesterase*?

It is an enzyme, which breaks down (for recycling) the *acetylcholine* neurotransmitter, so that it stops excitation of a nerve.

B 35. *Fibrinogen* is stored in the liver; True or false?

True; Fibrinogen (Factor I) is a glycoprotein, which is

involved in blood clotting, after being converted into fibrin, by thrombin.

B 36. What poisonous gas, on inhalation, turns the blood bright red?

Carbon monoxide, which gives the false impression that arterial blood is properly oxygenated.

B 37. What term describes excess fluid in the lungs?

Pulmonary oedema, caused by...

- ☠ Congestive heart failure

- ☠ Pneumonia

- ☠ Toxicity

- ☠ Medication reactions

- ☠ Low partial pressure of air (altitude)

- ☠ Trauma to the chest

B 38. How does vasoconstriction effect blood pressure?

It increases blood pressure. Vasoconstriction is the realisation of Boyle's Law, where reduction in space causes an increase in pressure.

B 39. *Oliguria* is defined as urine output of less than 1 litre a day; True or false?

False; less than 400 ml/day - for adults. Investigation is necessary, because there could be a serious underlying cause, particularly relating to the kidneys.

B 40. The prefix "adeno" refers to the liver. True or false?

False, it refers to the glands.

B 41. Giving the patient a hypotonic fluid will cause the cells to lose fluid; True or false?

False; The lower tonicity of the extracellular fluid will cause intracellular fluid to enter the cells, by osmosis.

B 42. An abnormality of the blood clotting process is known as a *coagulopathy*. True or false?

True.

B 43. What is the difference between *hypoxia* and *hypoxaemia*?

Hypoxaemia means there is an abnormally low level of oxygen (< 60 kPa) in arterial blood. Hypoxia means a reduced level of oxygen at the tissue level.

B 44. Why should an elderly patient, with a peptic ulcer, and mild pain, not be prescribed an NSAID?

NSAIDs are contraindicated for peptic ulcers, and the elderly.

B 45. What are the main causes of post-operative fluid depletion?

☠ Pyrexia ☠ Diuretics ☠ Drain losses

B 46. What is an *adhesion*?

An abnormal joining of tissues which, very often, can complicate the surgical site, particularly during laparoscopic cases.

B 47. What is the term to describe the product of stroke volume and heart rate.

Cardiac output: The volume of blood which the heart pumps through the circulatory system in one minute.

B 48. The suffix -*itis* signifies pain. True or false?

False, it refers to inflammation.

B 49. What does the *vagus nerve* do?

The vagus nerve is part of the *rest and digest* system and, as such, takes part in parasympathetic functions, connecting the brain with the neck, heart, lungs, and abdomen. The nerve is involved with the sense of taste, and provides sensory information between the brain and heart, lungs, abdomen, and throat. The vagus nerve also governs heart rate, digestion, and respiration.

B 50. Describe *diabetes insipidus.*

The condition where a patient produces copious amounts of urine, whilst experiencing pronounced thirst. Not to be confused with the more common *diabetes mellitus.*

B 51. What is *vasopressin?*

The anti-diuretic hormone (ADH), made in the hypothalamus and distributed by the posterior pituitary gland, which acts to retain extracellular volume by increasing water reabsorption in the kidneys. Additionally, it causes vasoconstriction and, consequently, increases blood pressure. Pharmacological ADH is used to treat *diabetes insipidus.*

B 52. Sodium is the principle ion (electrolyte) in intracellular fluid; True or false?

False; it is the main cation (positive ion) in extracellular (interstitial) fluid. The main intracellular ion (cation) is potassium.

B 53. In what body part or function does the *lock and key* mechanism occur?

Lock and key describes the "fitting" of a substance (ligand), such as a neurotransmitter, to its target receptor, such as a nerve cell.

B 54. What are the three types of extracellular fluid?

Plasma, Lymph, and Transcellular fluid (*cerebrospinal* and *synovial*).

B 55. Describe the term *extravasation*.

The discharge, or leakage, of fluid from the extracellular fluid compartment into surrounding tissue. Extravasation may also describe the shift of cells out of a blood vessel, during an inflammatory episode.

B 56. What is *eclampsia*?

When a pregnant pre-eclampsia patient develops convulsions, whilst suffering high blood pressure.

B 57. What does *extracorporeal* refer to?

Occurring outside of the body, such as with dialysis, perfusion, and *extracorporeal membrane oxygenation*, where a machine takes over the functions of the heart and lungs, by infiltrating the blood with oxygen.

B 58. Define *vasoplegia*.

Low systemic vascular resistance and hypotension, resulting from conditions such as sepsis, shock, and anaphylaxis.

B 59. Intracellular fluid represents what fraction of total body fluid?

① One quarter

② One third

③ One half

④ Two thirds

Answer: ④, Two thirds

B 60. Why can a patient, in septic shock, simultaneously suffer from too much and too little blood clotting?

Because they are experiencing *disseminated intravascular coagulation*, where blood clotting proteins are overly active, and block smaller blood vessels with small clots. The excess clotting depletes the store of platelets and clotting factors, with the result that excessive bleeding occurs in other parts of the body.

B 61. If a post-operative gastric patient is unable to feed, normally, how do they receive sustenance?

A patient may not be able to feed using the normal route of "mouth to digestive organs", for reasons such as intestinal obstruction, an inability of the small intestine to absorb nutrients, or other digestive organ dysfunction. In such cases, the patient will receive sustenance by *Total Parenteral Nutrition* (TPN), which is a method of feeding which bypasses the gastrointestinal tract and, instead, delivers nutrients intravenously, usually via a central line port.

TPN contains all of the fat, protein, glucose, vitamins, minerals, electrolytes, and trace elements (zinc, manganese, etc) which the patient needs.

B 62. If a patient is subject to an *apheresis*, what does it involve?

It is the extraction of specific components of the patient's blood, such as platelets or white blood cells.

B 63. What term describes a build-up of cholesterol, fat, and calcium on the walls of arteries?

Atheroma, or plaque. As the plaque/atheroma builds up, the internal diameter of the arteries is reduced, and the arterial walls become hardened. The resulting reduced blood flow can lead to stroke, myocardial infarction, and vascular disease.

B 64. How does "crenation" affect the cells?

They shrink, because of water moving out of the cell, into the interstitial space. This is caused by the osmotic effects of the interstitial fluid being hypertonic, with respect to the intracellular fluid. Crenation is what occurs after drinking sea water, which has a higher tonicity (more salt content) than the 0.9% weight/volume value of normal body fluid.

B 65. What is the principle neurotransmitter of the parasympathetic nervous system?

Acetylcholine (ACh), which acts on muscarinic and nicotinic (also part of sympathetic system) receptors. The functions of the parasympathetic system are often described by "SLUDD", which is an acronym for Salivation, Lacrimation, Urination, Digestion, Defecation. Muscarinic receptor activation causes a decrease in heart rate, relaxes blood vessels, constricts the airway, increases secretions and motility of the gastrointestinal tract, increases lacrimal and sweat gland secretion, and constricts the sphincter of the iris. Nicotinic receptors are involved in activation of muscle contraction, and are the target for neuromuscular blocking agents, such as atracurium, which prevents ACh from functioning, by binding with those nicotinic receptors and, thereby, blocks ACh from them (receptors).

B 66. The normal (adult) lactate range, per litre is:

---

① 0.5 - 1

② 1 – 1.5

③ 1.5 - 2

④ 2 – 2.5

Answer: ①   0.5 – 1. (Levels are higher for children)
Note: Some authorities claim that 0.5 – 1.5 is normal.

B 67. Where are *baroreceptors* located, and what is their function?

Nerve endings, located in the carotid sinus (neck) and aortic arch, that detect arterial flow and pressure changes, and send messages to the central nervous system to correct any imbalances in blood pressure.

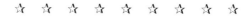

Pharmacology

P 1. Atropine is one of the emergency paediatric drugs; True or false?

True. Bradycardia can occur very quickly in children, and Atropine is an appropriate anticholinergic, because it is quick acting.

P 2. What are the stages of the *WHO analgesic ladder*?

Step	Description	Examples
1	Non-opioids	Aspirin, Paracetamol,

		NSAIDs
2	Weak opioid, with or without non-opioids	Lidocaine, Codeine, Oxycodone, Tramadol
3	Strong opioids	Morphine, Fentanyl

P 3. What is a *Depolarising Neuromuscular Block*, and how is it created?

Depolarization of skeletal muscles, making the muscle fibre resistant to further stimulation by acetylcholine. Suxamethonium is a quick acting depolarising neuromuscular blocking drug, typically used in Rapid Sequence Intubation.

P 4. What are the actions of *antimuscarinic* drugs?

Inhibition of acetylcholine on muscarinic receptors, in the parasympathetic nervous system. Actions include: relaxing smooth muscle, decreasing saliva secretions and sweat. Example drugs include Atropine, Hyoscine (Scopolamine), and Glycopyrrolate.

P 5. What is the *arm-brain circulation time*?

The time it takes an intravenously administered drug to travel from the hand/arm to the brain; Typically, less than one minute.

P 6. Induction agents usually cause an increase in systemic vascular resistance; True or false?

False, they usually reduce resistance, with consequent decrease in blood pressure.

P 7. What agent could a cardioversion patient be given, for treatment of an arrhythmia?

Amiodarone: 300 mg over one hour.

P 8. A substance which triggers a response, such as when a neurotransmitter binds with a receptor, leading to an effect, is known as an antagonist. True or false?

False; it is an *agonist*.

P 9. Why does suxamethonium cause *fasciculations*?

Suxamethonium depolarises muscular tissue, resulting in muscle contractions.

P 10. Atropine is an *agonist* for the acetylcholine neurotransmitter; True or false?

False; it is a competitive *antagonist* for muscarinic (acetylcholine) receptors.

P 11. What is *anticholinesterase*?

An agent which breaks down acetylcholinesterase, which

would otherwise decompose the acetylcholine neurotransmitter. Neostigmine is the typical anticholinesterase used to "reverse" a patient from perioperative non-depolarising neuromuscular paralysis.

P 12. How does *Archimedes Principle* concern reconstitution of a powdered drug?

The drug (solute) adds a some volume (displacement volume) to the solution, producing a volume which is greater than the volume of solvent used to produce the solution. For example, if 100 mg of a drug has a displacement volume of 0.3 ml (cc), and enough solvent is added so that the formed 100 mg solution is 1% weight/volume, then 9.7 ml solvent should be added, giving 100 mg in 10 ml.

P 13. A vasopressor increases blood pressure by constricting blood vessels; True or false?

True; it vasoconstricts. Examples: Adrenaline (Epinephrine), Metaraminol, Phenylephrine, and

Vasopressin.

P 14. What is an example dose of lipid emulsion, when treating local anaesthetic toxicity:

A bolus of 20% emulsion, 1.5 ml/kg, given over one minute. {As with all drugs, dosage information is constantly changing, so latest formulary entries should always be consulted}

P 15. What are the symptoms of opioid overdose?

- Pin-point pupils
- Slow respiratory rate
- Sighing
- Hypercapnia, then hypoxia

P 16. What is added to Noradrenaline (Norepinephrine) to prevent oxidisation?

5% dextrose.

P 17. How do non-depolarising neuromuscular blocking agents compete with acetylcholine (ACh), at the neuromuscular junction?

They bind with nicotinic ACh receptors, thereby blocking ACh from binding with the receptors, so preventing polarisation and resultant action potentials.

P 18. The suffix *-pril* signifies a sedative True or false?

False; it signifies antihypertensive drugs, such as *Ramipril*.

P 19. What does a Vagolytic drug do?

It inhibits the vagus nerve (*Cranial nerve X*). Examples are Atropine and Glycopyrrolate (Robinul).

P 20. Why is Ranitidine (or Zantac) given to the patient prior to caesarian section?

To reduce stomach acid, which might otherwise be regurgitated.

P 21. How many reversals are there for Propofol (Diprivan)?

None. Propofol has a short (5-10 minutes) metabolic half life, so reversal is by time.

P 22. Propofol (Diprivan) causes less respiratory depression than other induction agents; True or false?

False – it causes more respiratory depression.

P 23. Select 6 contraindications for Propofol.

a. Abnormal Metabolism of Fats

b. Epileptic Seizure

c. Hardening of brain arteries

d. Hypotension

e. Low blood volume

f. Tachycardia

g. Tachypnoea

h. Weakness

Answer: a, b, c, d, e, h.

P 24. What is a common antagonist for opiates?

Naloxone (Narcan).

P 25. What are the main side effects of Morphine?

- Nausea

- Respiratory depression

- Bradycardia

- Constipation

- ♠ Hallucinations

- ♠ Urinary retention

- ♠ Dry mouth

Note: Naloxone may be given as an antagonist.

P 26. Which opioid has the shortest half life?

Remifentanil (5 min); consequently, recovery is quick.

P 27. What is a *hyperbaric* drug?

One which occurs at higher than normal pressure or density, e.g., glucose added to Marcaine, as used in Caesarian Sections, so that the density of the local anaesthetic exceeds that of the cerobrospinal fluid; thereby allowing control of the spread of the drug by using patient position to utilise gravity.

P 28. What effect has Clonidone on blood pressure?

It lowers blood pressure – by vasodilation.

P 29. Why might a patient be given Vitamin K?

To antagonise the anticoagulation effects of Warfarin. Vitamin K aids blood clotting.

P 30. Ketamine gives sedation and analgesia; True or false?

True. Also, increases cardiac output, blood pressure, and heart rate, but does not depress the respiratory system, which is why it is useful in emergencies, when it is preferable to keep the patient breathing spontaneously.

P 31. What does *Naloxone* do?

Antagonises depression of the central nervous system, caused by opioids.

P 32. What is a typical perioperative use of Glycopyrronium (Glycopyrrolate, Robinul)?

To treat bradycardia. If the patient has a lot of secretions, glycopyrrolate may be given prior to anaesthesia.

P 33. Adrenaline (Epinephrine) is a vasodilator; True or false?

False; it is a vasoconstrictor - increases blood pressure.

P 34. Neostigmine is an example of a *respiratory stimulant*; True or false?

False; Neostigmine is an *anticholinesterase*. An example of a respiratory stimulant is Doxapram Hydrochloride.

P 35. A post-surgical patient, who is breathing room air, and using Morphine from a Patient Controlled Analgesia device, experiences a drop in oxygen saturation. What is the most likely cause?

Morphine induced hypoventilation.

P 36. What is the standard antagonist for opioids?

Naloxone, which counters the depression of the central nervous system, caused by opioids.

P 37. *Non Steroidal Anti Inflammatory Drugs* are contraindicated in kidney disease; True or false?

True; Also Stomach ulcers, Liver disease, Diabetics, and Pregnancy.

P 38. Select six contraindications to Glycopyrrolate:

  a. Allergies

  b. Cardiac issues

  c. Obesity

  d. Urinary problems

  e. Bowel problems

  f. Glaucoma

  g. Peptic ulcer

  h. Hypertension

Answer: a, b, d, e, f, g.

P 39. What is Sodium Bicarbonate typically used for?

Mixed with water, it can be ingested to reduce stomach acid, by increasing pH.

P 40. Define *first pass metabolism*.

When some drugs are taken enterally (via digestive system), the digestive system and liver will metabolise some (or all) of the drug, before it gets into the main circulation. As a result, the bioavailability of the drug is less than 100%. Agents, which are administered intravenously, do not suffer first pass metabolism, which means that they have a bioavailability of 100%.

P 41. If a patient has overdosed on a benzodiazepine, such as Midazolam, what can be given in way of an antagonist?

Flumazenil.

P 42. What is the significance of a pre-surgery patient who has been taking Aspirin?

The anti-platelet action of Aspirin could be a factor in surgery, due to the possibility of excessive bleeding.

P 43. Atracurium produces a depolarising neuromuscular blockade; True or false?

False; it is a non-depolarising drug.

P 44. Does Adrenaline (Epinephrine) cause bronchodilation or bronchoconstriction?

Bronchodilation.

P 45. A drug with high lipid solubility has a longer duration of action (generally) than a drug with a low lipid solubility; True or false?

False; a low solubility drug, such as Morphine, has a

longer effect because it takes more time to cross (leave) the blood-brain barrier.

P 46. Doxapram is an *analeptic* drug; True or false?

True; it stimulates the nervous system.

P 47. What does an *Antinicotinic* agent do?

It blocks cholinergic transmission between motor nerve endings and nicotinic receptors at the skeletal muscle neuromuscular junction. Used for non-depolarising neuromuscular blockade.

P 48. Atracurium interferes with normal neurotransmission; True or false?

True, it prevents acetylcholine from binding with motor end-plate receptors.

P 49. What is Balanced Salt Solution used for?

Irrigation in opthalmic surgery.

P 50. Noradrenaline (norepinephrine) causes peripheral blood vessels to dilate; True or false?

False; noradrenaline increases blood pressure, by constricting peripheral vessels.

P 51. What does *antitussive* agent do?

a. Prevent bleeding

b. Prevent coughing

c. Prevent spasms

Answer: b, Prevent coughing.

P 52. What is an *excipient*?

An excipient is an inert (inactive) substance, which helps deliver a product in a more suitable form. For example: a binding agent in a drug, to stop it from falling apart, to aid in delivery by adding lubrication, or to enable metabolism within a specific time period.

P 53. State the formal classification system for drugs?

The *Anatomical Therapeutic Chemical* (ATC) classification system, developed by the World Health Organisation. The ATC system categorises drugs with five levels of discrimination, based on the drug's:

- Anatomical target

- Therapeutic or pharmacological group

- Pharmacological, chemical, or therapeutic group

- Pharmacological, chemical, or therapeutic subgroup

- Chemical constitution

P 54. What is an **aliquot** sample?

A fraction of a supplied amount. For example, if a 20 ml syringe contains 10 mg of a drug, and the patient will need 2.5 mg boluses, splitting the 20 ml dose into 4 different 5ml syringes means 4 aliquots of 5 ml.

P 55. How is a drug **triturated**?

Meaning 1: The process of reducing the size of powdered particles, by grinding with mortar & pestle.

Meaning 2: The dilution of a powdered drug with an inert substance, such as powdered lactose.

P 56. What term describes a sudden reaction to an intravenous drug that has been administered too quickly?

Speed Shock: Signs include headache, flushing, chest tightness, irregular pulse, and cardiac arrest. Speed shock may be prevented by use of an infusion device.

Respiration & Circulation

C 1. The best way to open the airway of a patient with spinal injury is a *head tilt and chin lift*; True or false?

False; A spinal injury patient (or potential spinal injury) should not suffer movement which may aggravate their injury. Use a *jaw thrust* instead.

C 2. The intravenous infusion flow rate of blood can be increased by warming the blood; True or false?

True; heat reduces the blood's viscosity, making it flow more easily.

C 3. After removal from a fridge, what is the maximum time before blood must be used.

Four hours, if left out of the fridge.

C 4. Where does internal respiration occur?

In the tissues; it is the diffusive exchange of gases between the tissues and blood.

C 5. What are the main causes of tracheostomy obstruction?

Occlusion due to secretions – wet or dry. Suction may fix the problem. Otherwise, either the inner tube or the whole tube assembly may have to be replaced.

C 6. Why should a giving set be changed after a blood transfusion?

To reduce the possibility that drugs or incompatible fluids could rupture residual blood cells in the set, downstream of the mesh filter, and which might then be infused into the patient.

C 7. Select seven blood transfusion reactions from the following:

1. Back pain

2. Chills

3. Dark urine

4. Fever

5. Skin flushing

6. Blue lips

7. Confusion

8. Fainting

9. Shortness of breath

Answer: 1, 2, 3, 4, 5, 8, 9.

C 8. When transfusing blood, why should a pressure bag not be inflated to a pressure greater than 250 mmHg?

A higher pressure may cause cells of the transfusing

product to rupture and pollute the patient's bloodstream.

C 9. What is the main way in which a blood giving set differs from a standard intravenous giving set?

A blood giving set contains a 170-200 micrometer mesh filter, to prevent infusion of clots and redundant cells from the supplied product bag.

C 10. Select six signs of airway obstruction:

   a. Tracheal tug
   b. Aggression
   c. Intercostal recession
   d. Cyanosis
   e. Increased temperature
   f. Increased respiratory effort
   g. Stridor
   h. Cardiac arrest

Answer: a, c, d, f, g, h.

C 11. The trachea is anatomical dead space; True or false?

True – it does not take part in gas exchange, it is part of the airway conducting zone, not the respiratory zone.

C 12. *Anoxia* means no oxygen reaching the alveoli; True or false?

False – it is an absence of oxygen to the tissues.

C 13. *Fresh Frozen Plasma* is indicated in major haemorrhage; True or false?

False; it is indicated for coagulation of significant bleeding, but not major haemorrhage.

C 14. What is an anti-hypoxia device?

An interlinking system (hypoxic guard), electronic or mechanical, between oxygen and nitrous oxide flow controls, which ensures that the patient, being ventilated, does not receive nitrous oxide, without also receiving at least 21% oxygen. Anaesthetic practitioners must test these devices before every list.

C 15. What is the difference between type 1 and type 2 respiratory failure?

Respiratory failure means lack of oxygen in the blood – hypoxaemia.

Type 1: Hypoxaemia without hypercapnia.

Type 2: Hypoxaemia with hypercapnia.

C 16. Define blood *perfusion*?

The passing of oxygenated blood through a vessel or over an organ. A capillary receives oxygen by perfusion.

C 17. What is the significance of *capillary refill* time?

It provides an indication of the patient's peripheral perfusion and, possibly, whether or not the patient is hypovolaemic.

C 18. What is *Continuous Positive Airway Pressure*?

In spontaneous ventilation, non-invasive CPAP maintains positive airway pressure until the end of expiration. The closing pressure holds open the alveoli, so that partial pressure of arterial oxygen (pO2) and ventilation are improved.

C 19. Describe *Sellick's Manoeuvre*.

Application of pressure to the anterior arch of the Cricoid cartilage, to occlude the lumen of the oesophagus (upper end), preventing aspiration of stomach contents into the lungs. Typically used during *Rapid Sequence Induction*. A light force is required when the patient is drowsy, and 30-40 Newtons (3-4 kg) when unconscious.

C 20. What is a *Hypoxic Guard*?

A mechanical or electronically governed interlink between an anaesthetic machine's oxygen and nitrous oxide flow controls, which prevents the patient from receiving pure nitrous oxide, and maintains a ratio of, for example, 1:3 between oxygen and the nitrous oxide. If the oxygen flow falls below 200 ml/minute (200 cc/minute), the nitrous oxide flow shuts off.

C 21. One disadvantage of using a Laryngeal Mask Airway, over bag/valve ventilation, is that of its increased possibility of insufflating the oesophagus, and consequent gastric distension; True or false?

False – it is a reduced possibility.

C 22. CO_2 decreases as ventilation increases; True or false?

True. More gas exchange blows the CO_2 from the system.

C 23. What is the common term to describe paradoxical chest and abdomen movement?

See-saw. During anaesthesia, see-saw breathing is often a sign of upper airway obstruction.

C 24. Which of the following are causes of apnoea?

a) Residual effects of narcotic premedication.

b) Residual effects of anaesthetic induction or maintenance agent.

c) Advanced age.

d) Hypercapnia.

e) Severe hypotension.

f) Suxamethonium apnoea.

g) Pseudo cholinesterase.

h) Hypocapnia (no stimulus to breathe).

Answer: a, b, d, e, f, g, h.

C 25. What is a *pulmonary embolism*?

An obstructed pulmonary artery, caused by an embolus, typically originating from a deep vein thrombosis. Treatment might be anti-coagulation, by intravenous injection, or oral delivery.

C 26. What are the body's three principal types of circulation?

Pulmonary: Takes de-oxygenated blood from the right side of the heart, to the lungs, via the pulmonary arteries, and driven by the right atrium and ventricle. The blood then picks up a fresh supply of oxygen, from the alveoli, and transports the oxygenated blood to the left atrium, via the pulmonary veins.

Coronary: The arteries and veins which supply blood to the heart cells.

Systemic: The arterial system which transports blood from the left heart to the remaining parts of the body, and the venous system which returns the blood to the right heart.

C 27. Define *Central Cyanosis*.

A blue discolouring in the lips, tongue, and facial skin, typically caused by underlying respiratory and/or cardiac pathology, which allows poorly oxygenated blood to enter the arterial circulation.

C 28. Define *V/Q ratio.*

The value which describes the relative volumes of air reaching the alveoli (V = ventilation), and the flow (P = perfusion) of blood to the tissues specifically, the volume of air divided by the volume of blood flow.

V/Q > 1 Ventilation of blood is more efficient than perfusion: air is being loaded into the alveoli, and oxygen into the blood, but the circulation is not adequately transporting the oxygen to the tissues.

V/Q < 1 The opposite of the above: perfusion may be adequate, but the blood does not receive the proper amount of oxygen from pulmonary circulation.

V/Q = 0 (Shunt) Blood flows from the venous to the systemic circulation without being oxygenated by the usual pulmonary circulation and ventilation process.

A theoretical normal V/Q value is 1, but 0.8 – 0.9 might be more commonly encountered.

C 29. Describe the *Bohr* effect.

The binding affinity which oxygen has to Hb (haemoglobin), described by the oxygen-Hb dissociation curve. When the partial pressure of arterial CO_2 ($paCO_2$) increases, and pH lowers, Hb molecules tend to offload oxygen molecules to the tissues, and replace them with Hydrogen cations (H^+), thereby acting as a H^+ buffering system, which is part of the body's homoeostasis system, with respect to "normalising" pH.

C 30. What is a *Spirometer* used for?

To measure lung capacity, efficiency, and to diagnose respiratory problems, such as asthma and COPD.

C 31. What is the difference between *ventilation* and *oxygenation*?

Ventilation is the transfer of respiratory gases between the gas supply and lungs, whilst oxygenation refers to the process of supplying the tissues with oxygen.

C 32. What term describes an uncomfortable and abnormal pattern of breathing?

Agonal breathing, which is a type of desperate gasping, often mistakenly thought to be real breathing when, in fact, the patient is not ventilating, but in cardiac arrest.

C 33. Where does *external respiration* occur?

The lungs – gas exchange between the alveoli and blood.

C 34. What is the *second gas effect*?

When nitrous oxide is added to an anaesthetic gas induction regime, its rapid uptake by the surrounding capillary space produces an increased concentration of the accompanying inhalational agent.

C 35. What does the acronym *ARDS* stand for?

Acute Respiratory Distress Syndrome, which is a life threatening pulmonary oedema, caused by fluid in the alveoli, which results from lung inflammation.

Symptoms include low oxygen saturation, shallow breathing, fatigue, shortness of breath, and confusion.

C 36. How can a blood clot in the leg result in cardiac arrest?

If the clot detaches, it will travel through the circulation and, if it becomes lodged in an artery of a lung, it becomes a pulmonary embolism, blocking circulation to the heart, with consequent cardiac arrest.

C 37. What is the function of a *portal vein*?

A "normal" vein transports blood towards the heart, via the vena cavae. A portal vein gathers blood, which has drained from one or more organs, towards another organ. The *hepatic portal vein*, for example, takes venous blood from the digestive organs, gallbladder, pancreas, and spleen, and transports it to the liver.

C 38. What is a *varix* vein?

A *varix*, or *varicose*, vein is an unusually dilated

superficial (near the skin surface) vein, which has assumed a twisted course, is usually occurs in the legs, and is caused by faulty one way valves in the vessel. Arteries and lymph vessels may also become varicose, but varicose veins are more commonly found.

C 39. What is a Thorpe tube, and where is it used?

A vertically calibrated flowmeter - a device which governs the flow rate of a gas, at a constant pressure, and has a "bobbin" which floats up to a mark on the tube, corresponding with the particular flow rate, set by a rotary dial. Thorpe tubes are used to supply oxygen to facemasks on spontaneously breathing patients.

C 40. What function does *surfactant* provide?

Reduces surface tension between two surfaces, thereby reducing friction or cohesion. Pulmonary surfactant prevents the alveoli from collapsing, which might otherwise occur, during expiration.

C 41. What does "the patient has *atelectasis*" mean?

{*Atelectasis*: incomplete expansion} The alveoli do not fill with air, causing them to collapse, resulting in tachycardia, chest pain, cyanosis, and breathing difficulty. **Obstructive (resorptive)** atelectasis, the most common type of atelectasis, occurs when an airway is blocked (solids, tumour, blood, ...), preventing air from reaching the alveoli which, after giving off oxygen to the bloodstream, suffer reduced pressure, collapsing the alveoli. **Non-obstructive** atelectasis types include: pneumothorax, pleural effusion, **adhesive** (lack of surfactant), supine position, and **compression** atelectasis (exterior pressure on the lungs).

C 42. How can atelectasis be caused by anaesthesia?

When breathing 100% O_2 (oxygen), the O_2 diffuses from alveoli to bloodstream faster than oxygen can replenish the alveoli, causing a vacuum, which collapses the alveoli, in a condition called **absorption atelectasis**.

C 43. How does pulmonary oedema differ from atelectasis?

Atelectasis is the collapse of empty alveoli; pulmonary oedema is when the alveoli fill with blood or other liquid.

C 44. If the anaesthetist develops difficulty in ventilating an intubated patient, how might he/she determine if the problem is with the patient, rather than the circuitry?

By manually bagging the patient. Difficult bagging means the problem is with the patient (obstruction, atelectasis, etc); if bagging is easy, the problem is with the ventilation settings, breathing circuit, ET tube, etc.

C 45. What does FFP mask type mean?

Filtering Face Piece: Masks that protect against smoke, dust, and aerosols (aqueous fog), but not gas or vapours. FFP1 offers the least protection; FFP3 provides the most.

Anaesthetics

A 1. What is a *Bodok seal*?

A metal rimmed o-ring, which provides a gas tight seal between a high pressure gas cylinder and the connecting indexed pin fitting, as featured on an anaesthetic machine.

A 2. Why would deep extubation be used?

It reduces the chance of coughing - but does not prevent laryngospasm.

A 3. What Mapleson breathing circuit classification is a *bag-valve-mask* (Ambu bag)?

C - the reservoir bag is in the limb carrying fresh gas flow (afferent limb) to the patient.

A 4. A high cardiac output can reduce anaesthetic induction time; True or false?

False; the opposite is true. More blood is involved in uptake of the alveolar gas, per unit of time, so the blood is less concentrated, and equilibrium of pressure between the blood and alveolar space takes longer to achieve.

A 5. Why is nitrous oxide so quickly eliminated from the body?

Because it has very low blood and lipid solubility.

A 6. Induction agents can reduce cardiac output; True or false?

True.

A 7. An obese patient should receive oxygen through a nasal cannula, during the intubation process; True or false?

True; it provides NODESAT (*Nasal Oxygen During Efforts Securing A Tube*), which is the attempt to extend the safe apnoea time.

A 8. When an intubated patient is being ventilated, the APL valve has no effect; True or false?

True; the APL functions only under spontaneous (bag) mode.

A 9. What is the purpose of an *Aintree Intubation Catheter*?

Non-traumatic endotracheal tube exchange, and aiding

fibreoptic intubation.

A 10. Select six indicators for successful endotracheal tube insertion...

  a. Absence of fasciculations

  b. Tube condensation

  c. Auscultation of lungs (bilateral sounds)

  d. Sats of 95-100%

  e. Good end tidal CO_2 trace

  f. Visualisation of tube through vocal chords

  g. Auscultation of the stomach (no breath sound)

  h. Symmetrical chest rise

Answer: b, c, e, f, g, h.

A 11. A dose of muscle relaxant must be given, prior to insertion of a supra-glottic airway device; True or false?

False. Muscle relaxant is only necessary for intubating the patient.

A 12. During a rapid sequence induction, should different people apply different levels of pressure to the cricoid?

Yes; the application of 30 Newtons of force is distributed differently for different finger tip sizes; the larger the finger tip, the smaller the pressure.

A 13. What does MAC refer to, and what does it mean?

Minimum Alveolar Concentration: The concentration of an anaesthetic agent (as a % of one Standard atmosphere), in the alveoli, which would prevent response to a standard surgical stimulus, in 50% of a particular population of patients, and for a particular inhalational agent.

A 14. Does MAC reduce or increase with age?

Reduces.

A 15. What does a volatile agent's MAC number refer to?

The partial pressure, as a percentage of one atmosphere, to

produce the *Minimum Alveolar Concentration* level, for that particular agent, and class of patient. If, for example, the MAC number is 2, then 50% of subjects will fail to react to a standard surgical stimulation, when the agent produces an alveolar partial pressure of 15.2 (2% of 760) mmHg.

A 16. What is the Thyromental distance?

From the thyroid notch to the tip of the jaw. Less than 2.8 inches (7 cm) indicates possible difficult intubation.

A 17.   How often should an anaesthetic machine's oxygen failure alarm be checked?

Weekly.

A 18. After receiving a spinal anaesthetic, the obstetric patient starts to experience breathing difficulty, tingling in the fingers, hypotension, and bradycardia. What could be the reason?

A high spinal block, which should be countered by stopping the epidural (if present), tilting the mother onto the left side, giving 100% oxygen, and close monitoring

A 19. Before anaesthetic induction, how is the patient's *functional residual capacity* increased?

By pre-oxygenation, and sitting the patient up.

A 20. Spinal anaesthesia can cause vasoconstriction; True or false?

False; it causes vasodilation.

A 21. If an endotracheal tube is inserted too deeply, which bronchus is it more likely to enter?

The right (main) bronchus, which is more in-line with the trachea than the left.

A 22. What is *Backward Upward Right Pressure*?

BURP: Movement (Back, Up, patient's Right, Pressure) of the thyroid cartilage, to help visualisation of the vocal cords when intubating.

A 23. What effect, if any, has nitrous oxide on blood pressure?

Generally, none, or a little increase at the most.

A 24. What is *suxamethonium apnoea*?

The prolonged effects of suxamethonium, which means that when the patient reverses from anaesthesia, they might remain paralysed. As the patient becomes aware, blood pressure and heart rate increase, and the patient may start to sweat. A nerve stimulator will reveal that the patient is still paralysed, in which case, they should be re-anaesthetised and ventilated. The usual cause is the inability of the patient to metabolise suxamethonium.

A 25. What is *syncope*?

A temporary loss of consciousness.

A 26. What is a **TAP** block?

Local anaesthesia to the anterior and lateral abdominal wall, to provide analgesia.

A 27. How does obesity affect anaesthesia?

The airway can be "difficult", volatile agents take longer to reach equilibrium, and there is greater risk of aspiration.

A 28. What does *respiratory recruitment* refer to?

A transient increase in pulmonary pressure, with the aim of holding open the alveoli, to aid ventilation.

A 29. Hyperventilation causes high levels of CO_2 in the blood; True or false?

False; this term describes higher than normal rates of gas exchange, which means a higher rate of expelling the CO_2.

A 30. Why can't nitrous oxide be used as a sole anaesthetic agent?

Because it has a MAC greater than 100, which means it can never reach the level which produces anaesthesia.

A 31. What does *safe apnoea time* refer to?

The period, at induction, between when the patient stops breathing, and when the oxygen saturation drops below 90%.

A 32. What is the aim of *apnoeic oxygenation*?

A method of oxygenation, using nasal specula, to prolong *safe apnoea time*. During apnoea, more oxygen leaves the alveoli than is replaced by carbon dioxide, resulting in a low pressure which draws in air from the atmosphere, providing a passive ventilation.

A 33. Why would a patient need *Transnasal Humidified Rapid-Insufflation Ventilatory Exchange*?

THRIVE is a method of increasing safe apnoea time, for potential difficult airway cases, by fitting the patient with a trans-nasal oxygen device, having a flow rate of 70 litres of oxygen per minute. The intention is to passively oxygenate the patient until a definitive airway is realised.

A 34. What significance, to anaesthesia, is a patient with GORD?

Gastro-oesophageal reflux disease means persistent acid reflux. Intubation (RSI) protects the airway, but reflux may occur before induction, or at extubation.

A 35. What is the function of an *Adams Regulator*?

It reduces the high pressure gas, from a cylinder to the anaesthetic machine, to 12 psi (84 kPa).

A 36. Where, on an anaesthetic machine, is an interlink system?

The anti-hypoxia device is an interlink between the oxygen and nitrous oxide flows.

A 37. A *Bier Block* is a type of local anaesthesia; True or false?

False; It is a regional anaesthetic technique.

A 38. Describe the Bonfils intubation equipment.

A rigid retromolar intubation fibreoptic scope, with a straight shaft, and 40 degree curved tip, used in difficult airway cases, such as Pierre Robin syndrome.

A 39. What is the *sternomental* distance?

An assessment method to predict difficult intubations. For an adult, difficulty is anticipated if the distance between the upper manubrium (connects clavicles with sternum) and the point of the chin (mouth closed and head fully extended) is measured at less than 5 inches (12·5 cm).

A 40.   A large neck circumference is an indicator for difficult intubation; True or false?

True. Also:

- Short neck
- Receding mandible
- Protruding teeth
- Poor view of uvula
- Less than 5" (12.5 cm) sternomandibular distance
- Less than 35° neck extension

A 41. What is an *Electromyographic Endotracheal Tube*?

An ET tube, used in thyroid surgery, which allows monitoring of the Recurrent Laryngeal Nerve, with the aim of avoiding nerve damage.

A 42. Epidural means inside the *Dura Mater*; True or false?

False; it means **outside** the Dura Mater.

A 43. Describe *fluid challenge.*

The test for fluid responsiveness, where the patient is given 500 ml of fluid over 10 minutes. If the test is positive, it means the patient has a *preload reserve,* which suggests that further fluid administration will produce an increased cardiac output.

A 44. Explain *diffusion hypoxia.*

When a patient is emerging from N_2O (nitrous oxide) anaesthesia, large quantities of the N_2O cross from the blood into the alveoli (down its concentration gradient) and so, for a short period, the O_2 and CO_2 in the alveoli are diluted by the N_2O. This could cause the partial pressure of oxygen to decrease to the extent that hypoxia results.

A 45. One disadvantage of a RAE tube is that it cannot be used with a bougie; True or false?

False; the RAE tube can be straightened to allow passage of the bougie.

A 46. For what type of surgery would a Polar endotracheal tube be used?

Nasal intubation for maxillofacial surgery.

A 47. For long term use, an endotracheal tube with a low pressure cuff would be most suitable; True or false?

True. A high pressure cuff might restrict blood flow to the surrounding tissue, resulting in tissue necrosis.

A 48. The larger the internal diameter of an ET tube, the more resistance to gas flow; True or false?

False; a larger diameter means less resistance.

A 49. What is the formula to calculate paediatric ET tube size?

4 + (age / 4).

A 50. An anaesthetic machine's flow meter has an adjustable pressure wheel; True or false?

False; the pressure is constant, but the flow rate can be controlled.

A 51. If an intubated patient is administered N_2O (nitrous oxide), the ET (endotracheal) tube's cuff might suffer a decrease in pressure; True or false?

False; N_2O can cause an increased cuff pressure.

A 52. What is the ASA rating for a patient with a mild systemic disease?

ASA II.

A 53. What is an *Adjustable Pressure Limiting Valve*?

An expiratory relief valve, on an anaesthetic machine or portable breathing circuit, which governs Positive End Expiratory Pressure in spontaneous breathing.

A 54. What is the main pipeline gas supply pressure?

Approximately 4 bar, or 60 p.s.i., or 400 kPa, relative.

A 55. Describe the *second gas effect*.

The process whereby, when N_2O (nitrous oxide) is given with a volatile inhalational agent, at induction, the low solubility of the N_2O causes it to rapidly diffuse to the alveoli which, in turn, produces an abrupt increase in the concentration of the volatile agent, in the alveoli.

A 56. Explain how analgesia differs from anaesthetics.

Analgesia is pain relief, without loss of feeling, movement, or consciousness. **Anaesthesia** is loss of sensation, with or without consciousness.

Monitoring

M 1. A pulse oximeter gives an accurate indication of ventilation; True or false?

False; it measures the fraction of arterial haemoglobin which is saturated with oxygen. Ventilation refers to exchange of gases between the lungs and atmosphere (or breathing supply).

M 2. Define *hypercapnia*.

The increased level - > 45 mmHg (6 kPa) - of carbon dioxide in arterial blood, causing acidity, over stimulation of the respiratory centre, and depression of the central nervous system. Symptoms include lethargy, headache, hypertension, and confusion. Treatment is by assisted ventilation.

M 3. What is a typical postoperative adult fluid requirement?

Crystalloid: 30 ml/kg/day. A hypovolaemic patient may need more fluid, to normalise their fluid balance, and signs of hypovolaemia should be part of "Recovery" monitoring...

- Tachycardia of 90+ per minute

- Systolic blood pressure below 100 mmHg

- Capillary refill time > 2 seconds

- Respiratory rate > 20/minute

- Cool peripheries

M 4. What is shown on a *capnometer*?

The numerical presentation of expired carbon dioxide level. A typical (adult) range is 35 - 40 mmHg, or 4.7 – 5.3 kPa.

M 5. What is *Pulse Pressure*?

The difference between systolic and diastolic pressures. If BP is 120/80, pulse pressure is 40 mmHg. If pulse pressure is greater than 60 mmHg, in older patients, they might be at risk of cardiovascular disease, or heart valve regurgitation. A narrow pulse pressure of < 25 mmHg might be an indicator of congestive heart failure.

M 6. An ECG trace reflects muscular activity of the heart; True or false?

False, an electrocardiogram detects electrical activity.

M 7. What is *bradycardia*, and how is it treated?

Slow (brady) heart (cardia) rate. An antimuscarinic, such as Glycopyrronium, can be used to counter bradycardia.

M 8. Name some causes of *tachycardia*.

Anaemia ☠ Fever ☠ Hypovolaemia ☠ Myocarditis ☠ Pain ☠ Vasodilatio ☠ Vagolytic drugs ☠ Anxiety

M 9. An *International Normalised Ratio* value for a patient, who is taking Warfarin, should be between 0.8 and 1.2; True or false?

False; that is the range for a healthy person, not on Warfarin. For the Warfarin patient, the range is 2 – 2.5.

M 10. A shark fin capnograph is one sign of bronchospasm; True or false?

True. Also, wheezing, prolonged expiration, increased airway pressure (during IPPV), reduced tidal volume.

M 11. What is the normal range of arterial blood pH?

7.35 – 7.45. Lower than 7.35 indicates acidity, and greater than 7.45 means an alkaline condition.

M 12. What is indicated by an arterial blood gas with:

- Low pH
- Low CO_2

☞ Low HCO3

Answer: Metabolic (low HCO3) acidosis (low pH) with respiratory compensation (low CO2).

M 13. What does a shark fin capnograph, in an anaesthetised patient, signify?

Possible airway obstruction, such as bronchospasm.

M 14. What is the normal blood glucose level, for a Type 1 diabetic?

On rising: 5-7 mmol/litre (90-126 mg/dL).

After meals: 5-9 mmol/litre (90-162 mg/dL).

Other times: 4-7 mmol/litre (72-126 mg/dL).

M 15. A *central line* cannot be used to deliver rapid fluid infusion; True or false?

False – it **can** be used for rapid infusion.

M 16. Pulse oximetry is the best indicator of airway compromise; True or false?

False; it can take several minutes for the blood oxygen level to fall – a change in CO_2 is a more immediate indication of ventilation issues.

M 17. What could be the causes of a patient's increased fluid loss?

Infection ☠ Fever ☠ Diarrhoea ☠ Vomiting ☠ Diuretics ☠ Kidney problems

M 18. If a patient has a left sided pneumothorax, on which side will there be breath sounds?

The right side.

M 19. Name some of the patient assessment factors of a Surgical Recovery Practitioner.

☑ Consciousness level

- ⊞ Oxygen saturation

- ⊞ Pulse rate/force/rhythm

- ⊞ Respiratory rate

- ⊞ Blood pressure

- ⊞ Temperature

- ⊞ Blood glucose

- ⊞ Skin colour

- ⊞ Pain control

- ⊞ Postoperative nausea/vomiting management

- ⊞ Pressure area management

- ⊞ Fluid balance

- ⊞ Other outputs: drains/wounds/stoma/NG tube

- ⊞ IV patency

- ⊞ Dressing patency

M   20. What is the purpose of *Thromboelastography*?

TEG tests the efficiency of blood coagulation, platelets, fibrinolysis, and clot strength.

M 21. What are the primary symptoms of fluid losses?

- ⚲ Hypotension

- ⚲ Tachycardia

- ⚲ Oliguria (low urine output)

- ⚲ Confusion

M 22. What is the origin of the term *B.M.*, with respect to testing of blood sugar levels?

The test was developed by, and named after, the **Boehringer Mannheim** Pharmaceuticals company – now called Roche.

M 23. What standard monitoring device indicates *atrial fibrillation* (AF)?

The ECG (electrocardiogram) - the P wave is usually absent in AF.

M 24. What are the symptoms of *hypercapnia*?

☞ Confusion

☞ Drowsiness

☞ Dizziness

☞ Headache

☞ Dyspnoea (short of breath)

☞ Lack of patient cooperation

M 25. What is the purpose of a *central venous catheter*?

☒ Continuous measurement of blood pressure

☒ Measures vascular tone

☒ Measures circulating blood volume

☒ Long term access for drug administration

☒ Parenteral nutrition

☒ Hydration

☒ Specimen collection

M 26. What does a *Bi Spectral Index* measure?

Depth of anaesthesia, using the patient's EEG (electroencephalogram) activity.

M 27. What are the symptoms of *hypoxaemia*?

Confusion ◆ Tachycardia ◆ Tachypnoea ◆ Sweating ◆ Wheezing

M 28. What are the symptoms of *tension pneumothorax*?

- ☞ Hypotension
- ☞ Distended neck veins
- ☞ Tracheal deviation (opposite pneumothorax)
- ☞ Tachypnoea
- ☞ Tachycardia
- ☞ Chest pain
- ☞ Expanded chest
- ☞ No pulse
- ☞ Muffled heart and lung sounds

M 29. How is *cardiac output* measured?

CO is the product of stroke volume and heart rate.

M 30. What is *Beck's Triad*?

The principle indicators of cardiac tamponade:

- ☞ Hypotension OR narrow pulse pressure
- ☞ Jugular venous distension
- ☞ Muffled heart sounds

M 31. What effect could air bubbles in an arterial line tubing have on the pressure reading?

Some of the pressure will be taken up by the process of compressing the air, rather than being applied to the transducer pressure sensor (Wheatstone Bridge), resulting in damping of the waveform, and an inaccurate arterial pressure reading. The tubing, itself, does not absorb any of the pressure, because it is incompressible.

M 32. What part of the cardiac cycle is represented by the *QRS complex*?

Depolarisation of the ventricles.

M 33. What does a *Sequential Organ Failure Assessment* (SOFA) score indicate?

It quantifies the degree of organ failure, in the septic patient, using various clinical parameters, such as blood pressure, respiratory rate, and Glasgow Coma Score.

M 34. How does a *QSOFA* score differ from *SOFA*?

The quick SOFA scoring system is a simpler and less comprehensive method of determining sepsis, in ICU, where one point is given for each of the following:

- Low blood pressure (Systolic BP $\leq$ 100 mmHg)
- High respiratory rate ($\geq$ 22 breaths/min)
- Glasgow coma scale < 15.

Any two of theses parameters provide a definition for possible sepsis.

M 35. How is *Cardiac Index* (CI) measured?

By dividing the patient's cardiac output by body surface area, giving a value of *litres/minute/square metre*.

M 36. Restlessness and agitation are earlier signs of poor ventilation than cyanosis; True or false?

True. Cyanosis can take several minutes to form, so is not a dependable indicator of ventilation problems.

M 37. What is the normal adult urine output?

400-500 ml/day, which suggests adequate kidney function.

M 38. If an arterial line transducer is raised to a higher level than the patient's phlebostatic axis, will the pressure reading show:

(a) An incorrectly lower value

(b) An incorrectly higher value

(c) The correct value

Answer: (a) Lower, because the "head of fluid" in the transducer line has been reduced.

M 39. Convert 4 mmol glucose to mg/dL.

Multiply the mmol by 18, to give 72 mg/dL (18 * 4).

M 40. What are the main categories of *tachycardia*?

Tachycardia type	Impulse source
Atrial (supraventricular)	Atria
Sinus	Sinus node
Ventricular	Ventricles

M 41. What is considered to be the most common complication during the post-anaesthesia period?

❂ Airway problems

- Pain control

- Infection

- Nausea and vomiting

Answer: Nausea and vomiting are the most common, with airway issues, such as obstructions, being the second most common type of complication in the post anaesthetic phase.

M 42. List some of the signs of internal haemorrhage.

Hypotension	"Bruising"
Dizziness	Blood in the urine
Pain: abdomen or chest	Dizziness
Nausea/vomiting	Clammy skin
Breathing difficulty	Headache
Thirst	Clammy skin

M 43. What is the definition of *hypovolaemia*?

A reduction in the normal level of blood volume; typically between 10% and 20% below normal.

M 44. What are twinned heart beats called?

Answer: Bigeminy.

M 45. What acid-base condition is signified by **pH** = 7.27, **HCO3-** = 18, **pCO2** = 35 mmHg?

pH is acidaemic, and bicarbonate (**HCO3-**) is acidic, so this is a metabolic acidosis, with partial compensation from the respiratory system, where low **pCO2** is due to hyperventilating in the attempt to raise pH towards the normal range of 7.35 – 7.45.

M 46. What are the two types of metabolic acidosis?

Normal Anion Gap (NAGMA) and High Anion Gap (HAGMA) metabolic acidosis. NAGMA is due to loss of bicarbonate that is replaced with chloride. HAGMA is all other causes, such as excess ketones, excess lactate, toxins, or kidney failure.

M 47. What scoring system determines phlebitis at a peripheral cannula site?

The VIP Score, where 0 (no phlebitis) to 5 (treatment for thrombophlebitis and resite cannula) is a grading range.

☆ ☆ ☆ ☆ ☆ ☆ ☆ ☆ ☆

Surgery

S 1. What is a *closed reduction*?

A non-surgical manipulation and setting of a fractured bone, which does not involve cutting through the skin, and where the position is maintained by plaster cast. *Closed* refers to the fact that the skin is not opened (cut), as with *open* surgery, where the skin is dissected. *Reduction* means the broken ends of the bone are brought together, in proper alignment.

S 2. What type of procedure is a *panendoscopy*?

An endoscopic examination of the pharynx (pharyngoscopy), tongue, larynx (microlaryngoscopy), oesophagus (oesophagoscopy), and bronchi (bronchoscopy); and taking of biopsies.

S 3. Define *Empyema*.

The collection of pus from a cavity, such as the pleural space, where it is referred to as *pyothorax* or *purulent pleuritis*. Removing the empyema is achieved by needle drainage, or surgery.

S 4. Why would a *queckenstedt test* be undertaken during a lumbar puncture?

The test is used to verify the correct flow of cerebrospinal fluid, and absence of subarachnoid blockages, by applying pressure to the jugular vein, to increase the venous pressure. If there is a small or slow pressure increase, then the cause, such as tumour or vertebral intrusion, must be determined.

S 5. What type of instrument is a *trochar*?

A triangular edged instrument, with a sharp and pointed

end, which is fitted into a cannula for introduction into a blood vessel or body cavity, such as when introducing laparoscopic ports.

S 6. What does *percutaneous* mean?

Through the skin by, for example, forcing a needle through the skin to extract a substance, or to deliver an instrument or therapeutic agent.

S 7. What is the purpose of a *Harmonic scalpel*?

To cut or cauterise vessels by means of ultrasound energy (rather than electrical diathermy), which has the effect of less bleeding than occurs with steel scalpels.

S 8. What is the purpose of a *pigtail drain*?

The percutaneous drainage of fluid from a cavity (eg, pleural), duct, or abscess; fitted by Seldinger technique, with the pigtail end uncoiled, during placement. Once placed, a negative pressure of 20 cmH_2O is established, and a drain fitted. Radiology should confirm proper placement, and show that the pigtail has reverted to its pigtail shape. Frequent flushing might be needed if blockages are to be avoided.

S 9. What is an *apheresis*?

The extracorporeal (outside of body, through a machine) extraction of a specific blood component, such as platelets or cholesterol, with the remaining blood being returned to the patient. A commonly used apheresis procedure is *lipoprotein apheresis*, which is the extraction of low density lipoprotein (LDL) cholesterol from the blood of patients who are unable to control their cholesterol levels by normal means, such as diet.

S 10. What is the function of a *curette*?

An instrument, usually ring or scoop (like with ice cream scoops) shaped, to scrape away tissue or debris during an excision or biopsy, or during a cleaning process. *Curette* can also be used as a verb: to *curette* a body part.

S 11. What is an *Angioplasty?*

The percutaneous widening of a blood vessel, such as the coronary artery, by inflating a small balloon, to allow proper blood flow. If a *stent* (tubular mesh) is inserted, the procedure is referred to as *percutaneous coronary intervention*, or PCI.

S 12. What is the surgical term to describe the endoscopic removal of kidney stones?

Percutaneous Nephrolithotomy. A cystoscope is placed into the bladder, a tube is fed up the ureter, into the kidney, which then fills the kidney with a contrast dye, for easy viewing by x-ray. An endoscope and stone fragmenting tools are then passed into the kidney, from an incision in the back.

S 13. What type of bacteria is *Chlorhexidine* effective against?

Chlorhexidine gluconate is a broad spectrum disinfectant and antiseptic against gram positive and negative bacteria, and is used as a skin cleaner, and as a preparation for a surgical site.

S 14. What is a *backslab*?

A plaster cast, cut in two, to provide a "shelf" like support to a limb, with the open part allowing access to the limb.

S 15. When inserting a chest drain, where is it placed?

Thoracentesis: The tubing is placed into the pleural space, and the collection vessel is placed at a lower atmospheric level than the chest, to allow drainage by pressure gradient.

S 16. A colostomy is an opening made between the colon and what else?

The abdomen; The opening in the abdomen wall is called a *stoma*, where the end of the bowel connects with a colostomy bag, which is outside the body.

S 17. What is an *abdominal aortic aneurysm*?

A dilation of part of the aorta, within the abdomen. The aneurysm usually does not cause any symptoms, unless it ruptures, which is more likely if the aneurysm is more than 2″ (5 cm) in diameter (double normal size). When aneurysms do rupture, fatality is very likely. Men over the age of 65 are at most risk of having an abdominal aortic aneurysm.

S 18. Define *Insufflation*.

The filling of a body cavity with low pressure gas, such as carbon dioxide, during, for example, endoscopic procedures, to give surgeons a better view of the abdominal cavity.

S 19. How does an *evulsion* differ an *avulsion*?

Evulsion is the act of extracting or pulling something out, such as veins in varicose vein procedures. **Avulsion** means torn away, such as with an avulsion fracture, where a bone fragment becomes detached from the main bone, but is still attached to a ligament or tendon.

S 20. What is the purpose of a *ligature*?

To occlude or tie off a vessel, using an appropriate type of thread; typically used to prevent blood from leaving the vessel.

S 21. Define *curettage*.

Scraping tissue or debris from the inside of a hollow organ, using an instrument called a *curette*.

S 22. What is the name of the clamp which is used to occlude a blood vessel - to stop bleeding?

A haemostat (USA hemostat), which looks like a pair of scissors, but with a blunt nose, and toothed gripping parts. A more popular term is *arterial forceps*, which are available in different sizes.

S 23. When a patient is to have a procedure needing application of a tourniquet, when should antibiotics be given?

Before inflating the tourniquet cuff, otherwise the antibiotics will be prevented from reaching the exsanguinated surgical site.

S 24. What is a *cystogram*?

A procedure which allows the observation, assisted by x-ray, of the urethra and, how the bladder fills and empties. A catheter is passed through the urethra, into the bladder, wherupon a contrast dye is introduced.

S 25. What is a surgical *flap*?

A plastic surgery method of transferring tissue, such as skin and muscle from a recipient (flap) to a donor site, whilst maintaining an intact blood supply. If the flap is taken from a site adjacent to its target (recipient) point, then it is a *local flap*. If the donor flap comes from a different part of the body, it is termed a *free flap*.

S 26. What types of procedure would non-absorbable sutures be appropriate for?

For long duration tissue closure, such as for skin wounds; the repair of the bowel, blood vessels, and tendons. Non-absorbable sutures are either left in place permanently (internal), or are eventually removed by a clinician – usually if they are external sutures.

S 27. Nylon and Prolene are examples of synthetic non-absorbable sutures; True or false?

True. The body's own enzymes will absorb or dissolve the sutures, with absorption time dependent on the type of suture material.

S 28. Povidone-iodine (Betadine) contains iodine and what other main ingredient?

Detergent, which helps to loosen solidified detritus from the skin.

S 29. What is the purpose of a *chest drain*?

Inserted into the pleural space, it removes air, fluids, or pus. The external end of the tubing is attached to a bottle of water, to act as a seal against air leaking back into the pleural space.

S 30. If a surgical procedure name has the suffix "ectomy", what does it signify?

Removal of an organ, such as the appendix or tonsils.

S 31. What does *débridement* refer to?

The removal of debris - foreign matter, or contaminated or dead tissue - from a damaged or infected lesion, which prevents proper wound healing. After *débriding* the wound, healing can commence.

S 32. Define *effusion*.

The discharge or build-up of liquid, typically from a cavity. When excess fluid accumulates between the pleura (layered membranes) - "water on the lungs" - it may cause breathing difficulty, coughing, or pain.

S 33. A Jehovah's Witness patient is scheduled for a laparotomy; what special equipment might be required?

A Cell Saver, as an alternative to the potential need for blood transfusion.

S 34. What type of case is denoted by NCEPOD category 2?

A *National Confidential Enquiry into Patient Outcome and Death* category 2 case is one which is classed as "urgent", which means the patient needs surgery within hours of the decision to operate has been made.

S 35. In any procedure where surgical site infection is a high risk, such as orthopaedic cases, the ventilation system should be of a *turbulent* flow type; True or false?

False; *Laminar Flow* ventilation is considered the more effective type, although ongoing research questions the effectiveness of laminar flow systems. In theory, the laminar technique pushes pathogens down and out from the surgical field, making surgical site infection less likely than with turbulent flow ventilation.

S 36. What is meant by the term *evisceration*?

Displacing visceral (internal) tissue or organs from a body cavity, such as during transplantation.

S 37. What is the definition of surgical site infection?

The most general definition of an SSI is one where an infection develops withing thirty days of surgery, where no implant is made. Alternatively, if there is an implant, and an infection occurs within one year of surgery, it may also be classed as an SSI. A further classification is between incisional site and organ SSI.

S 38. What are the perioperative rules for infection control?

The generic principles are...

① Patients should bathe on the day of their surgery.

② Hair should be cut with clippers – not razors.

③ Skin to be disinfected immediately prior to incision.

④ Prophylactic antibiotics should be given one hour before surgery.

⑤ The patient should not be cooler than 34° C, before anaesthesia.

⑥ Surgery should comply with aseptic protocols.

⑦ A minimum number of people in the theatre.

⑧ Wounds to be dressed with interactive dressings.

S 39. During post-surgical recovery, a patient is equipped with a PCA (patient controlled anaesthesia) device, which does not deliver any analgesia unless the patient requests (button press) it, and a "lock-out" period has expired; True or false?

False; a PCA may be programmed to deliver a continuous infusion, in addition to a patient triggered bolus (push), known as a *background infusion*.

S 40. What are the methods for repairing an abdominal aortic aneurysm?

∞ Open surgery: an abdominal incision is made to access the aorta, and the aneurysm repaired with a graft.

∞ Endovascular repair: a less invasive and traumatic procedure, where the aneurysm is accessed via a catheter in the groin, and a stent and graft passed up through an artery to the damaged area.

S 41. What are the main methods of managing intraoperative bleeding?

∫ **Vascular occlusion**: The haemorrhaging vessel is occluded, with clamps or clips, then closed by ligation (sutured).

∫ **Packing**: The wound site is packed and tamped with swabs, until a more permanent repair is made, or the wound heals itself.

S 42. What is the name of the process of using a balloon to widen an artery?

Angioplasty. To make a widening permanent, a stent (mesh tube) is fixed into the widened section.

Angio indicates a blood vessel, and *plasty* signifies some sort of shaping or structural modification.

S 43. What type of solution has a solute content which dissolves in water?

An aqueous solution, such as a crystalloid. The solute is hydrophilic with water, which means the solute's molecules "merge" with the water molecules, forming a new substance.

S 44. If a patient needs pus, air, or liquid removed from the pleural space, what common technique is used?

Thoracentesis, which is chest drainage by needle aspiration. After numbing the insertion site with a local anaesthetic, a needle is passed through the chest to the pleural space, possible guided by x-ray or ultrasound. Once the pleural space has been reached, the unwanted substances are aspired through the needle.

S 45. What is the name of the process of squeezing blood from a limb, distal to proximal?

Exsanguination, such as before a tourniquet is applied, in regional anaesthesia for a lower limb procedure.

S 46. How is the process of increasing the space in a vessel, hollow organ, or opening to an organ described?

Dilatation - to dilate – as with urethral dilatation and upper GI (gastrointestinal) endoscopy and dilatation.

S 47. What does *necrotic* tissue refer to?

Tissue that has experienced necrosis, which is when some of a tissue's cells have died, due to toxins, disease, inflammation, or failed blood supply. If a large part of the organ is necrotic, it is termed *gangrene*. Necrotic tissue is irreparable, and must be surgically removed, either by debridement, or amputation.

S 48. What is *biosurgery*?

Aka *Larval Debridement Therapy*: The use of maggots to remove necrotic tissue. The maggots eat the dead or infected tissue, but not healthy tissue, and they stimulate healing by releasing substances to destro bacteria.

S 49. What oral prophylactic is given immediately before intubation for an emergency caesarian section GA?

Sodium citrate, 30 ml, an antacid, as a defence against acid aspiration.

S 49. What is a *Fistula*?

An abnormal passage (hole or tissue connection) between organs, or between a cavity and the body surface, often caused by severe inflammation of, for example, part of an intestine. Extended childbirth can also cause fistulas, such as between vagina and bladder. Surgery can also be the cause of a fistula, especially in urology procedures.

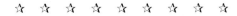

Books by John England

📖 **Glossary of Anaesthetics**
http://amzn.eu/g4Ah8AO

📖 **Blood Gases**
https://www.amazon.co.uk/dp/B09755Pd1F/ref

📖 **Q & A: Anaesthetic Principles, Volume 1**
http://amzn.eu/iIbr8eK

📖 **Q & A: Anaesthetic Principles, Volume 2**
http://amzn.eu/4eKMyRe

📖 **Q & A: Anaesthetic Principles, Volume 3**
http://www.amazon.co.uk/dp/B0876F7V6S

📖 **Q & A: Anaesthetic Principles, Volumes 1-3**
https://www.amazon.co.uk/dp/B087BJ7YXW

📖 **Q & A: Basic Life Support**
http://amzn.eu/acoxDel

📖 **Pass Your Drug Calculation Test**
http://amzn.eu/duk6uT7

📖 **Basic Drug Calculations**
http://amzn.eu/d0SWt0c

📖 **Drug Calculation Workbook**
http://amzn.eu/d39gtl3

📖 **Drug Calculation Examples**
http://amzn.eu/76zGfkJ

📖 **Drug Calculations By Formula**
http://amzn.eu/eW9SEg3

📖 **Advanced Drug Calculation Workbook**
http://amzn.eu/7zDyFQh

📖 **Nurse Q & A: Anatomy and Physiology**
http://amzn.eu/f6nRC6G

📖 **Q & A: Respiratory System**
http://amzn.eu/7RqNNxa